Asthn

How To Get Asthma F

By

Vicki Joy

Other Books by Vicki Joy

ACNE: Natural Acne Scar Treatments for Clear Skin
http://amzn.to/29WlzA4

ANTI-AGING: The Anti-Aging Guide to Healthy Skin and the
Fountain of Youth
http://amzn.to/1Q1P5CU

ANXIETY: Getting Free From Fear And Panic Attacks
http://amzn.to/1Thj2uS

ARTHRITIS: How to Relieve and Reverse Rheumatoid Arthritis
Today
http://amzn.to/2a8bmLf

Unstoppable You! How to Build Your Confidence and Go After
the Life of Your Dreams
http://amzn.to/2hhpwSw

FOCUS: The Key to Success
http://amzn.to/1rQsG0H

INTROVERT: How To Use The Introvert Advantage And
Introvert Power
http://amzn.to/1XV8WH9

RELAXATION
http://amzn.to/1TTY6JM

WEIGHT LOSS - The Mindfulness Diet
http://amzn.to/1V6XMN7

circumstances will any legal responsibility or blame be held against the publisher for any reparation, damages, or monetary loss due to the information herein, either directly or indirectly.

Respective authors own all copyrights not held by the publisher.

The information herein is offered for informational purposes solely, and is universal as so. The presentation of the information is without contract or any type of guarantee assurance.
The trademarks that are used are without any consent, and the publication of the trademark is without permission or backing by the trademark owner. All trademarks and brands within this book are for clarifying purposes only and are the owned by the owners themselves, not affiliated with this document.

Table of Contents:

1. Introduction

2. What Is Asthma?

3. What Causes An Asthma Attack?

4. Asthma and Diet

5. Natural Remedies for Asthma

Introduction

Thank you so much for downloading *"Asthma - How To Get Asthma Free Naturally"*. This book contains proven steps and strategies on how to overcome asthma.

Over 20 million people in the United States can't take breathing for granted because they are suffering from a chronic respiratory ailment called asthma.

The lungs are made up of hollow tube-like structures which divide into branches which further divide into smaller branches. The branches get smaller and smaller till they end is small pockets where the blood takes the oxygen from and leaves carbon dioxide. In asthma patients, the hollow tubes become inflamed and swell up making it difficult and very uncomfortable for them to breath. Exercise, stress, humidity, pollution, medication and allergens may trigger the asthma due to this inflammation.

Though asthma has no known cure, proper medication and changes in environment and way of living may help suppress and relief the symptoms and help those affected lead a more normal lifestlye. Some of the most common symptoms of asthma are coughing, chest congestion, wheezing, lack of breath, fatigue and anxiety. The symptoms may be varied for different persons. Asthma may be triggered by allergens, but there is also non-allergic asthma. The non-allergic asthma can be initiated or aggravated by factors like stress, climatic changes, exercise and other illness.

Managing asthma becomes a very critical and integral part of the lives of the people suffering from it. To do this, one has to be careful to keep away from things that affect the respiratory organs and take proper medication or home remedies as advised by a physician.

An asthma episode is the aggravation of the asthma symptoms. A severe asthma episode in called an asthma attack. During an asthma attack, the smooth muscles along the bronchial tubes start contracting and constricting the air passage, resulting in less flow of air. This further increases the inflammation causing swelling and constriction in the air passage. Due to lack of air, the cells in the air passage produce more mucus, which further exacerbates the constriction in the air passage. This lack of air causes the asthma symptoms.

Asthma attacks may vary from very severe to not so severe. In severe asthma attacks, the air passage constriction may be so effective that a medical emergency condition may result due to lack of oxygen reaching the vital organs. Severe asthma attacks can be fatal. The sensation during an asthma attack has been described similar to that of drowning by some sufferers.

Knowing the warning signs or mild symptoms of asthma can be lifesaving as it will caution the sufferer in time to take preventive measure. An inhaler or medication can be used in time to control the symptoms before they become too severe. There may be long phases of time between attacks, where a sufferer doesn't notice any symptoms or very few mild symptoms. But sometimes the symptoms may get aggravated and stay so for long periods of time.

Asthma can be passed on from generation to generation genetically. Children of parents with a history of asthma are 40 percent more likely to develop the ailment than kids without a genetic history of asthma. The genetic factor for asthma cannot be removed but the symptoms of this ailment are highly treatable. The rising numbers of asthma sufferers among children has become a cause of concern for many. There is a wide belief that exposure to allergens in early childhood may initiate asthma.

Change in environment and lifestyle is the best possible way to counter asthma. The common phrase 'prevention is better than cure' is apt when referring to asthma. Its better to avoid the triggering elements that initiate the symptoms of asthma. Various methods may be used to avoid specific allergens. Your home should be kept clean to avoid dust mites, pollen and animal dander that may trigger asthma. Pets and smoke are also common known triggers. To avoid pollen triggers, stay indoors as much as possible, and when outside, ride with windows up in the car. Dehumidifiers and air conditioners are also helpful for asthma sufferers on hot humid days.

Medications prescribed by a physician are an important weapon in the defense against asthma and its associated symptoms. To decrease the swelling in the lungs' tissue lining steroids are commonly prescribed, while bronchodilators are used to relax the air passage ways of the lungs to open them up. Steroids are long acting while the bronchodilators are short and fast acting. These medicines can be used in the form of pills or inhalers.

Though asthma symptoms vary from moderate to serious and asthma attacks can be fatal, asthma is also highly treatable. A proper asthma management action plan and correctly complimenting environmental and lifestyle changes with medication can make a healthy active life possible for a person suffering from asthma.

Thanks again for purchasing this book. I hope you enjoy it!

What Is Asthma?

Asthma is a respiratory disorder characterized by difficulty in inhaling and exhaling, wheezing, and coughing. It doesn't choose its victims. Whether you're a child or an adult, male or female, this health condition can make you run to your doctor. Though it was once considered as a harmless ailment, today it is one of the leading causes of hospitalization, especially among children. Not only that, but asthma medications rank as the second largest category of prescriptions written by doctors.

Asthma is one of the most common chronic diseases of childhood, affecting more than 6 million children. During an acute asthma episode, the airway lining in the lungs becomes inflamed and swollen. In addition, mucus production occurs in the airway and muscles surrounding the airway spasm. Combined, these cause a reduction in air flow.

Asthma is characterized by:

- Airway inflammation: the airway lining becomes red, swollen, and narrow.

- Airway obstruction: the muscles encircling the airway tighten causing the airway to narrow, making it difficult to get air in and out of the lungs.
- Airway hyper-responsiveness: the muscles encircling the airway respond more quickly and vigorously to small amounts of allergens and irritants.

Understanding the Different Types of Asthma

Traditionally, asthma is often classified into two types - intrinsic asthma and extrinsic asthma. However, as per the modern medical world, there can be so many different types of asthma, such as steroid-resistant asthma, occupational asthma, nocturnal asthma, exercise-induced asthma, intrinsic asthma, and allergic asthma. Besides that, doctors now use four basic classifications to determine the severity of asthma, including severe persistent, moderate persistent, mild persistent, and mild intermittent.

Allergic Asthma - More than 90% of the patients suffer from allergic asthma. This is the most common type, which can be diagnosed when asthma attacks are triggered by specific allergies. The good thing here is that such allergies are easily avoidable and identifiable if you get the treatment at the right time. So, make sure you contact your doctor immediately once you experience any such thing.

Intrinsic Asthma - This is one of the most common types of asthma that usually affect people aged 40 years and up. It does not normally occur in children. The cases where children have been affected by intrinsic asthma are rare. It is mainly caused by regular inhalation of irritating chemicals, such as cleaning products, smoke, and perfumes. It is not an easy condition to treat. Therefore, it is very important for you to be very alert and talk to your doctor about every symptom that you are experiencing that might be indicative of intrinsic asthma. The goal here is to to prevent the condition from worsening.

Exercise-Induced Asthma - This is also one of the common types of asthma and it occurs usually in people who practice heavy exercise on a regular basis. One of the important signs of this condition includes coughing fits caused by exercising heavily. When you work out heavily, your lungs lose necessary moisture and heat, which eventually results in asthmatic attacks and breathing difficulties.

Nocturnal Or Sleep-Related Asthma - In this type of asthma, the asthma symptoms occur in the patient during the night hours. The typical symptoms include coughing, wheezing, shortness of breath, and difficulty breathing. This can be a very serious situation especially for children who are experiencing this condition. You must consult your doctor immediately if you are being affected by this condition. Some common possible causes for nocturnal or sleep-related asthma include gastroesophageal reflux disorder, allergens in the lowered room temperature, and allergens in the bedroom.

Occupational Asthma - Occupational asthma has also become increasingly very common these days - probably because of the increased level of pollution in the air. This types of asthma occurs by prolonged exposure to allergens or industrial chemicals.

Inhalation of chemical fumes and dust is a major cause of these types of asthmatic attacks.

Steroid-Resistant Asthma - You are strongly recommended to take your medications as directed by the doctor. If you don't take medications as prescribed, of if you take an overdose of medication, you may be at the risk of developing a more serious condition, which is known as steroid-resistant asthma. In this case, the patient stops responding to the medications.

All these types of asthma require medical assistance regardless of their severity level.

What Causes An Asthma Attack?

Asthma triggers include allergens, irritants, or any other condition that cause your asthma symptoms to worsen. It's important to know what triggers your asthma symptoms. Triggers vary from person to person, so you should learn which specific ones affect you. While it may be impossible to avoid every single asthma trigger, there may be things you can do to limit your exposure to your specific triggers. To avoid or lessen the instances of asthma attacks, being able to identify and avoid your triggers is important.

There are many different kinds of asthma triggers. Triggers can be an allergic reaction to allergens that irritate the lungs. Some of the most common triggers are listed below.

Environmental Tobacco Smoke (Secondhand Smoke)
Environmental tobacco smoke is often called "secondhand smoke" because it is smoke that is breathed in not by a smoker but by a second person nearby. Parents, friends, and relatives of children with

asthma should try to stop smoking and should never smoke around a person with asthma. They should only smoke outdoors and not in the family home or car. They should not allow others to smoke in the home, and they should make sure their child's school is smoke-free.

Dust Mites

Dust mites are in almost everybody's home, but they don't cause everybody to have asthma attacks. If you have asthma, dust mites may be a trigger for an attack. Dust mites are microscopic creatures that feed on dead skin flakes and they thrive on areas like your bed, your bed-sheets, pillows and fabrics. As a result of dust mites in the home, asthma sufferers may end up wheezing, because of the dust mites present in the very clothes they are wearing or the beds they are sleeping on. To help prevent asthma attacks, use mattress covers and pillow case covers to create a barrier between dust mites and yourself. Don't use down-filled pillows, quilts, or comforters. Remove stuffed animals and clutter from your bedroom.

Flower Pollen

If you have an allergy to pollen or outdoor mold, allergy season can be tough on your asthma. And if you have multiple allergies, it also can be long and painful season. Tree pollen generally causes problems in early spring, grass pollen strikes in late spring and early summer, and weed pollen is active in late summer and fall. While you can't avoid pollen entirely, you may want to talk to your healthcare provider about whether the following tips may be helpful depending on your specific allergies:

- Try to keep your windows closed, and if possible, use air conditioning
- If possible, stay indoors with your windows closed during the late morning and afternoon hours, when pollen and mold-spore counts are highest

Outdoor Air Pollution

Pollution caused by industrial emissions and automobile exhaust can cause an asthma attack. Pay attention to air quality forecasts on the radio and television and plan your activities for when air pollution levels will be low, if air pollution aggravates your asthma.

Cockroach Allergen

Cockroaches and their droppings may trigger an asthma attack. Get rid of cockroaches in your home and keep them from coming back by eliminating their food supply. Cockroaches are usually found where food is eaten and crumbs are left behind. Remove as many water and food sources as you can because cockroaches need food and water to survive. Vacuum or sweep areas that might attract cockroaches at least every 2 or 3 days. You can also use roach traps or gels to decrease the number of cockroaches in your home.

Pets

Furry pets may trigger an asthma attack. When a furry pet is suspected of causing asthma attacks, the simplest solution is to find the pet another home. If pet owners are too attached to their pets or are unable to locate a safe, new home for the pet, they should keep the pet out of the bedroom of the person with asthma.

Pets should be bathed weekly and kept outside as much as possible. People with asthma are not allergic to their pet's fur, so trimming your pet's fur will not help your asthma. If you have a furry pet, vacuum often to clean up anything that could cause an asthma attack. If your floors have a hard surface, such as wood or tile, and are not carpeted, damp mop them every week.

Mold

When mold is inhaled or breathed in, it can cause an asthma attack. Get rid of mold in all parts of your home to help control your asthma attacks. Keep the humidity level in your home between 35% and 50%. In hot, humid climates, you may need to use an air conditioner or a dehumidifier or both. Fix water leaks, which allow mold to grow behind walls and under floors.

Strenuous Physical Exercise

For many years, it was believed that people with asthma should not or could not exercise. Today, healthcare providers recommend that most people, including people with asthma, get at least 30 minutes of moderate exercise most days of the week.

Follow the suggestions below to help eliminate or alleviate the likelihood of exercise on-set asthma:

• If your healthcare provider has prescribed medicine for asthma symptoms that may be triggered by exercise, be sure to take the prescribed medicine according to his or her instructions.
• Warm up by stretching or walking for about 10 minutes before you exercise
• Consider a cooling-down period as well.

Other Triggers

Some medicines; bad weather such as thunderstorms, high humidity, or freezing temperatures; and some foods and food additives can trigger an asthma attack. Strong emotional states can also lead to hyperventilation and an asthma attack. Learn what triggers your attacks so that you can avoid the triggers whenever possible and be alert for a possible attack when the triggers cannot be avoided.

Common signs and symptoms of an acute asthma episode include:

- Coughing
- Wheezing
- Breathlessness - while walking or while at rest
- Respiratory rate increased
- Chest tightness
- Chest or abdominal pain
- Fatigue, feeling out of breath
- Agitation
- Increased pulse rate
- Inability to participate in sports

During an acute asthma episode, signs and symptoms of increasing respiratory distress or breathing difficulty include:

- Inability to talk in sentences, using phrases or only words
- Retractions - increased use of chest, neck or abdominal muscles to breathe
- Refusal to lie down - a child may prefer to sit or lean forward in order to make breathing easier

It is important to remember that not everyone with asthma has the same symptoms.

Asthma and Diet

Although asthma is a breathing disorder there are certain foods which may both trigger asthma or prevent asthma from striking. Fortunately, if you maintain a good diet with plenty of fresh natural foods, you shouldn't have too many problems.

There are certain foods that will increase the likelihood of the onset of asthma symptoms. These foods should be avoided or limited if you suffer from severe asthma. Proteins, particularly animal proteins are one of the biggest culprits.

Try to determine which foods may be asthma triggers for you. When you first begin this program, in order to give yourself the best possible outcome, I recommend eliminating or at least significantly reducing certain foods from the diet for a week. After this time you can include them in your diet providing your symptoms are under control. Just be aware that certain foods are less friendly to your asthma condition.

Foods To Avoid For A Week

- All meats (Beef, Lamb, Goat, Chicken, Turkey, Pork, Bacon, Ham, Fish)
- All Dairy (Milk, Yogurt, Cheese)
- Eggs
- Limit Sugar Consumption (avoid Cakes, Cookies, Ice-Cream, Sweet Drinks, Chocolate)
- Alcohol & Drugs (Other Than Your Prescribed Medications)

Do not avoid protein altogether as it is an essential part of the diet which will help with growth, muscle repair and fighting diseases. There are many non-animal sources of protein, including vegetables (especially sprouts), nuts, seeds and grains.

Another important rule to live by would be, only eat when you are hungry and do not overeat. Overeating may cause you to hyperventilate. Overeating is also unhealthy for a number of other reasons so it shouldn't be a big surprise to hear that overeating is bad for your asthma too.

You should always eat only when you are hungry, your body will let you know when it is time to eat. Don't even eat when you first get out of bed if you aren't hungry. Wait until your body tells you that it is ready for food. If you have to take tablets in the morning, whether they are vitamins or medications, have a glass of water, tea, coffee or juice. When your body is ready for food, it will digest it much easier than eating eating you believe that you must eat at a particular time.

Superfoods For Asthma

There are a number of foods which are known to help asthmatics due to their anti-inflammatory properties, their impact on cardiovascular and general health. For optimum freedom from your asthma, it would be a good idea to get as many of these foods into your diet on a daily basis as possible.

Here are top 10 superfoods that work best:

1. Probiotics

2. Spices (Especially: Ginger, Turmeric, Liquorice, Black Pepper, Iodized Sea Salt, Mustard, Paprika, Cumin & Cloves)
3. Chlorella and Spirulina
4. Garlic/Onion
5. Chilli
6. Walnuts
7. Sprouted Vegetables
8. Green Apples
9. Green Vegetables
10. Coffee

Coffee may be a little controversial. Caffeine is known to cause hyperventilation, however it is also a very effective bronchodilator and has always worked for me. Moderation is probably the key. Everybody is different so I encourage you to find out what is going to work best for you. Plain old water is hard to beat too. You should be drinking sufficient quantities of water based on your weight and physical activity. Especially when consuming coffee. Coffee acts as a diuretic, which increases the excretion of water out of your body.

Probiotics

Probiotics are only now being discovered to prevent or eliminate many health complications including asthma. Probiotics are live microorganisms or friendly bacteria found in fermented foods. It can be found in fermented vegetables, yogurt, kefir or in capsules, powders or liquid supplements.

We are still in the early stages of our understanding, but new research in recent years is showing that by boosting our immune system, probiotics can help - considering asthma is an autoimmune disease. Probiotics have been proven to provide many health benefits and I would encourage you to research the benefits for yourself.

Supplementation

The amount of nutrition we obtain from our foods depends solely on the quality of the foods that we eat. Sometimes even with the very best intentions, we can experience malnutrition in some form simply because the nutrients we are seeking are not present in the foods we are eating.

Modern farming is a major factor in this. Soil condition is one factor. Another factor is that we don't eat fresh fruit and vegetables until days, weeks or even months after they have been picked. During this time, they are losing nutritional value everyday. To ensure we are getting all of the vital nutrients we need to sustain a healthy life along with being asthma free, a good idea would be take a supplement. A good quality multiple vitamin is your best strategy to defend yourself against malnutrition. Asthmatics especially need to ensure that they are not deficient in Vitamin D or B. These vitamins especially Vitamin D, are said to be important for the immune system.

Food Allergies

Foods, food additives and chemicals are not particularly common triggers for asthma; they only affect a small percentage of people with asthma who are susceptible to food allergies. They trigger asthma either as part of a food allergic reaction or a chemical intolerance.

It is important to understand how your own body responses to particular foods, because we are all different. Some of us have less to worry about, whilst some will have food allergies or intolerances which can be severe.

An allergy is when the body's immune system overreacts to a substance that is normally harmless to most people. These substances are also known as "allergens". Being exposed to an allergen may cause irritation or swelling in areas of the body such as the nose, eyes, lungs and air passages. A severe food allergic reaction is known as anaphylaxis and can be life threatening.

Natural Remedies for Asthma

The person suffering with asthma needs regular treatment for longer duration to bring the disease under control. Natural remedies may be a useful alternative for asthma sufferers. As always, it is advisable to follow the recommendations for your healthcare provider. There are many triggers and causes for asthma and they differ from one individual to another.

Allergies are assumed to be the biggest trigger for asthma attacks, but not everyone who has allergies may have asthma too. This disease can happen due to allergies, heredity, choked lungs, inflammation of respiratory passages and airways, blockages in nostrils, weather conditions and other irritants. These triggers can cause narrowing of the breathing track - especially the trachea - to cause problems in breathing.

Holy basil leaves have been shown to be a beneficial tool in preventing asthmatic attacks. Chewing a few holy basil leaves with honey first thing in the morning, or chewing holy basil leaves with rock salt or black pepper can stave off an coming asthmatic attack. Drinking tea made with holy basil leaves regularly helps the body in countering asthma due to allergies and the swelling of respiratory passages.

Another trusted natural remedy for asthma is consuming a paste made by mixing one teaspoon of turmeric powder in one tablespoon of honey. Turmeric has anti-inflammatory properties that are beneficial in relieving the inflammation in the airways for asthma sufferers, and by extension, provides relief for the feeling of tightness in the chest. Honey also has many anti-inflammatory and anti-allergic properties, in addition to strengthening the immune system. It can be added as part of the regular help manage asthma symptoms and soothe inflamed airways.

Half teaspoon of licorice roots mixed with a cup of water and boiled on a low flame for some time is another good natural remedy for asthma. Licorice is commonly used as a natural cough suppressant.

Another very effective natural remedy can be prepared by mixing one teaspoon of fenugreek seeds with 250 ml of water and boiled on a low flame till its volume is reduced to half, later adding one teaspoon each of ginger juice and honey with the mixture and consuming it every day is an excellent remedy for asthma. Ginger root and fenugreek seeds are known for the powerful anti-inflammatory properties, which can relieve inflamed respiratory passages.

Linseed may also provide an excellent natural remedy which can soften mucus and help relieve a dry cough. The relieving of a dry cough relieves asthma substantially. Take 20 grams of linseed and boil them on low flame with 300 ml of water till water is reduced to half, strain the mixture and add 10 grams of sugar in it. Sipping this mixture one teaspoon at a time in an hour is extremely effective.

There are certain precautions which a person can take to avoid or stave off an asthma attack, and these precautions also count as natural remedies. Dusting the bedroom daily or alternate days with a hepa vacuum cleaner will help in keeping allergens away to prevent an attack. Other precautions include:

- Avoiding using perfumes
- Covering mattresses with a plastic cover
- Washing bedding weekly in hot water (to kill dust mites)
- Avoiding using brooms for cleaning as this stirs up dust (vacuum instead)
- Wearing scarf will prevent hot and cold air from reaching and aggravating sensitive airways
- Avoiding dairy products, meat and greasy food which may be difficult to digest

Taking the above precautions will help in preventing or lessening the incidences of asthmatic attacks. Increased intake of apples, leafy vegetables, carrot and tomatoes have been shown to helps the body in countering triggers of asthmatic attack.

Below are other forms of natural remedies for asthma relief:

1. Mix a tablespoon of honey with a half a tablespoon of cinnamon powder and consume prior to sleeping. Or boil eight to ten cloves of garlic in half a cup of milk and consume it at night. This is a wonderful natural asthma remedy for those who are in the early stages of asthma.

2. Another helpful natural asthma remedy is figs, which help in draining phlegm. Soak three to four dry figs in water, then eat the soaked figs on an empty stomach along with drinking the fig-infused water.

3. Steeping ginger tea with minced garlic cloves may offer asthma relieve if taken two times in a day.

4. For asthma relief, mix one gram of dry ginger powder and one gram of black pepper in one teaspoon of molasses or honey.

5. Turmeric may be taken along with honey in the morning on an empty stomach to provide some asthma relief.

Benefits of Natural Remedies for Asthma

Asthma can be treated in a number of ways. Most commonly, asthma is treated with medications prescribed by a medical professional. These prescriptions should be followed and medications taken as prescribed. Natural remedies and precautions are ideal for avoiding asthma triggers and for reducing the number of asthmatic episodes, and in lessening the severity of attacks.

Below are some benefits of using natural remedies:

- Reduce or eliminate episodes of persistent coughing, difficulty breathing, or wheezing (especially in the morning), tightness in the chest, recurrent ear, nose and or throat infections (i.e. additional symptoms associated with the asthmatic condition)
- Reduce use or reliance on antihistamines, decongestants, nasal sprays, inhaled steroids, inhaled bronchodilators, antibiotics, cough, cold and flu remedies

- If you have a more advanced condition and if you have been repeatedly dissatisfied with the outcome of other treatment (or preventive) measures, you may benefit best from a combination of natural remedies that treat both sinus and bronchial symptoms of asthma and promote the body's own healing abilities naturally!

Conclusion

Thank you again for purchasing this book!

I hope this book was able to help you to understanding a bit more about asthma and some it the triggers that bring on asthmatic attacks. More importantly however, I hope that you were able to get some useful information about natural remedies that offer relief from the frequency and severity of asthma attacks.

The next step is to try out the natural remedies and other precautions covered in this book. Find the ones that works best for you, and use those as part of your arsenal for combating asthma and its triggers.

Finally, if you enjoyed this book, please leave me a positive review. I would greatly appreciate it!

Thank you and all the best!

Printed in Great Britain
by Amazon

82456581R00031